DITCH THE DIET LIFE

Ultimate Journal for Women who are Ready to Ditch their Diet Life & Create a Loving Marriage with Food

Created by:
BRITTNAE GIESAU

DITCH THE DIET LIFE

Copyright © 2018 Brittnae Giesau
BrittnaeG Publishing

All content is original work by Brittnae Giesau © 2018

Photography by Kayla Myers - Blaze Photography © 2017

Logo Creation by Shawna Poliz Design © 2017

Design template created & license released by *Canva.com*.

All rights reserved. No part of this book may be reproduced, scanned, or distributed in any printed or electronic form without permission.

ISBN-13: 978-0692985878

For more information email info@theblinggirldiaries.com.

In change there is fear.

In change there is discomfort.

These feelings are necessary.

These feelings are welcome.

I choose love & guidance in place of fear.

I will listen, accept & release all fear.

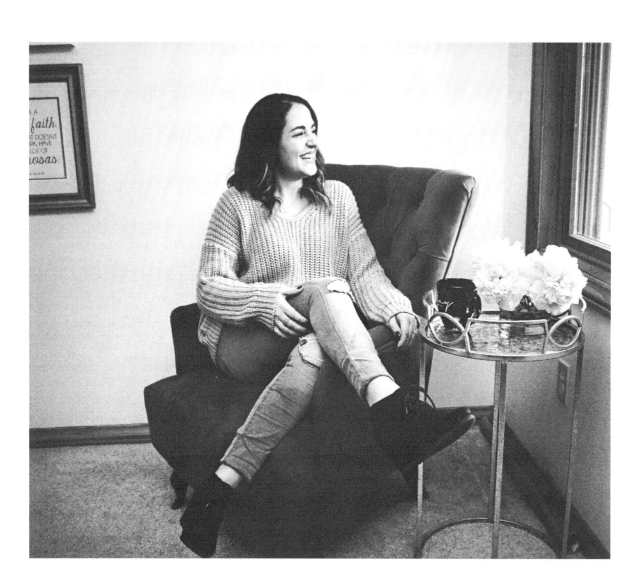

MEET BRITTNAE

Hey Gorgeous ~ I'm Brittnae, your *Ditch the Diet Life* expert. I am a health and wellness coach to the woman that may be battling emotional eating, riding the diet roller coaster, struggling to lose weight and unable to feel love for the body she is in. I have lived years in the diet cycle: binging, restricting, hating myself for something I ate, falling off the proverbial wagon because of one "bad" meal, and not knowing where to turn or which diet to try next. It wasn't until I began embracing the body that I am in and appreciating the woman in the mirror that I could truly live the life that I wanted without dieting.

This journal is not for the woman that wants to track her food calorie by calorie. This is for the woman that is tired of living a life ruled and run by her diet. The woman that wants to enjoy a plate of pasta and a glass (or 2) of Pinot Noir with the girls instead of worrying about six pack abs. This is for the woman that wants to begin living her life outside of a diet and still lose weight.

I am that woman. I created this journal to take the icky feelings out of food and fitness tracking and put love for yourself and your body back into a healthy lifestyle.

USING YOUR JOURNAL

The pages are not dated or outlined by day 1, 2, 3, etc. because I do not want you to feel as though you "missed" a day and have fallen behind. This is your journal to track the days, your way. What I don't want you to feel is that you had a "bad meal" and skip journaling your day because of it. The questions in this journal are designed to help you work through your feelings and reactions to meals to ditch your diet life.

Logging your food:
Feel free to track your food as you see fit: if you want to track by portions, go for it; if you want to track calories or macros, be my guest; if you simply want to say "bowl of veggies", awesome. This area is open to your interpretation. I do strongly urge you to allow yourself the leniency to step away from making it an obsessive counting process.

Rating your day & answering your questions:
Be *HONEST* with yourself. This process is about releasing yourself from a dieting mentality. If you are filling in the answers of things that you think you "should" be answering, you're not serving yourself. Be clear and honest with your answers without shame, guilt or fear.

Free Write:
The questions listed in the free write area, are items to assist you to spark a journaling habit. The free write area is just that: a FREE write. It is the time when you sit down, light a candle, turn on a little background music and write what is on your heart. You do not need to limit this just to your food and fitness. The questions are simply items you may want to address from your day, but feel free to use this space to journal anything that may be on your mind or heart.

BREAKDOWN OF FOOD

All food is protein, carbohydrates, fats, vitamins, minerals & water. You need all of these nutrients. Your body will break down and utilize them no matter what you eat.

Protein: Necessary for growth & repair of all tissues, hormone & enzyme function & regulation of fluids. Animal sources (chicken, eggs, dairy, fish, etc.) & vegan sources.

Carbohydrates: Preferred source of fuel for muscle & essential for brain function & breaking down into glucose for energy for the body. (Starches, Sugars, & Vegetables)

Fats: Provide essential fatty acids & a source of energy for the body, absorb fat-soluble vitamins, cell structure, regulate immune system, protect organs & blood pressure. Plant & animal sources as well as oils.

Vitamins: Refer to a dr. or specialist to find the vitamins best for your body.

Water: The body needs at least 48-64 ounces per day; don't wait until you're "thirsty" stay hydrated!

WHAT ARE YOUR FAVORITE PROTEIN SOURCES?

WHAT ARE YOUR FAVORITE CARBOHYDRATE SOURCES?

WHAT ARE YOUR FAVORITE FAT SOURCES?

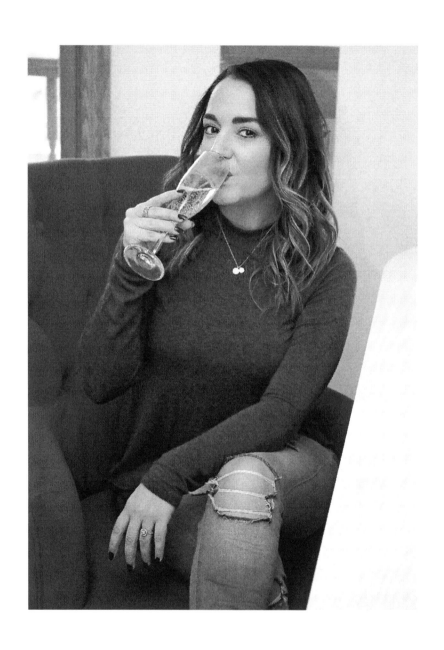

FINAL THOUGHTS

I hope that you enjoy this journey. Be gentle with yourself. Ditching your diet mentality is not going to happen overnight, it may often times creep back up on you. But what you're about to begin is a life changing process to love yourself and live in a healthier body built by mindset. Every 10 days or so you will have the opportunity to do a little check in. Ask yourself the hard questions, evaluate & celebrate how far you've come each time.

I am providing you with my social channels below so that you may contact me to connect, ask questions, and share your progress with me directly.

Also, please join the *Ditch the Diet Life* private online community by searching "ditch the diet life" on Facebook groups. Here you will be able to connect with other women that are journaling their process, finding freedom from their diet life, and build empowering relationships.

Now, lets turn the page and get started!

Facebook: http://Facebook.com/BrittnaeGiesau
Instagram: http://Instagram.com/Brittnae.Giesau
Twitter: http://Twitter.com/BrittnaeGiesau
Blog: www.TheBlingGirlDiaries.com

Join our private Ditch the Diet Life online community at http://facebook.com/groups/ditchdietlife

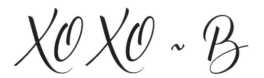

DITCH THE DIET LIFE

3RD DAY OF JANUARY, 2018

WORKOUT: 30 MIN. YOGA, 40 MIN LIFT

MEDITATION TIME: 15 MIN.

BREAKFAST: 2 EGGS WITH SAUSAGE & 1/2 BAGEL

LUNCH: SALAD W/CHICKEN & GREEK YOGURT DRESSING

DINNER: ROTINI PASTA IN RED SAUCE & ITALIAN SAUSAGE WITH BROCCOLI

SNACKS: APPLES & PEANUT BUTTER, SHAKEOLOGY

ALCOHOL: YES OR NO, HOW MUCH - YES ~ 1/2 GLASS OF RED WINE

ON A SCALE OF 1-10, HOW WOULD YOUR RATE YOUR DAY?

ABOUT A 7. I DIDN'T EAT OFF PLAN, BUT DIDN'T EAT ENOUGH TODAY TO FUEL MY LIFT WORKOUT

DID YOU EXPERIENCE ANY PHYSICAL REACTIONS TO SOMETHING YOU ATE?

CHEESE W/DINNER TURNED MY STOMACH A BIT THIS EVENING

WHAT WAS THE BEST THING ABOUT YOUR DAY? WHAT ARE YOU GRATEFUL FOR?

EVEN THOUGH I WAS BUSY I MADE SURE TO KEEP MY FOOD CHOICES ON MY PLAN. I AM GRATEFUL FOR GETTING BACK TO MY NORMAL SCHEDULE AFTER A BUSY HOLIDAY.

WATER CHECK: 1 2 3 4 5 6 7 (8)

Ditch the Diet Life ~ Brittnae Giesau

FREE WRITE

3RD DAY OF JANUARY_, 2018

HERE ARE SOME QUESTIONS TO ASK YOURSELF:
DID YOU FEEL ANY GUILT AFTER EATING SOMETHING TODAY? HOW IS THAT FEELING SERVING YOU? HOW MUCH OF YOUR DAY WAS SPENT THINKING ABOUT FOOD? WHAT IS AN EMOTION OR SITUATION CONNECTED WITH YOUR FOOD THAT YOU NEED TO LET GO OF TODAY?

I never really felt guilty for anything I ate today, but i definitely didn't eat enough. This is one of my downfalls when it comes to trying to eat on a plan. I spent so much time dieting over the years that eating MORE food is scary as hell for me. I'm always afraid that if I eat even though I'm not hungry at that moment that it's going to deter me from hitting my goals, even though I know that the goals that I want to hit require me to eat more food. Definitely soemthing that I'm still working on mentally. Today was the first day the kids went back to school since the Christmas break and it felt SO good to have my time back. I got a lot of work done this morning, had a little pampering nail appointment and started dinner earlier. I'm a creature of habit and need that shedule to feel normal!

I didn't really think about food today much because I was so busy, but I'm definitely letting go of feeling guilty and not going to shove food in my face tonight when i'm not hungry so I don't feel bad about it later. Tomorrow is another day!

DITCH THE DIET LIFE

_____ DAY OF _____, 20____

WORKOUT: MEDITATION TIME:

BREAKFAST:

LUNCH:

DINNER:

SNACKS:

ALCOHOL: YES OR NO. HOW MUCH

ON A SCALE OF 1-10, HOW WOULD YOUR RATE YOUR DAY?

DID YOU EXPERIENCE ANY PHYSICAL REACTIONS TO SOMETHING YOU ATE?

WHAT WAS THE BEST THING ABOUT YOUR DAY?
WHAT ARE YOU GRATEFUL FOR?

WATER CHECK: 1 2 3 4 5 6 7 8

Ditch the Diet Life ~ Brittnae Giesau

FREE WRITE

_____ DAY OF _____, 20___.

HERE ARE SOME QUESTIONS TO ASK YOURSELF:
DID YOU FEEL ANY GUILT AFTER EATING SOMETHING TODAY? HOW IS THAT FEELING SERVING YOU? HOW MUCH OF YOUR DAY WAS SPENT THINKING ABOUT FOOD? WHAT IS AN EMOTION OR SITUATION CONNECTED WITH YOUR FOOD THAT YOU NEED TO LET GO OF TODAY?

DITCH THE DIET LIFE

_____ DAY OF _____, 20____

WORKOUT: MEDITATION TIME:

BREAKFAST:

LUNCH:

DINNER:

SNACKS:

ALCOHOL: YES OR NO. HOW MUCH

ON A SCALE OF 1-10, HOW WOULD YOUR RATE YOUR DAY?

DID YOU EXPERIENCE ANY PHYSICAL REACTIONS TO SOMETHING YOU ATE?

WHAT WAS THE BEST THING ABOUT YOUR DAY?
WHAT ARE YOU GRATEFUL FOR?

WATER CHECK: 1   2   3   4   5   6   7   8

Ditch the Diet Life ~ Brittnae Giesau

FREE WRITE

_____ DAY OF _____, 20___.

HERE ARE SOME QUESTIONS TO ASK YOURSELF:
DID YOU FEEL ANY GUILT AFTER EATING SOMETHING TODAY? HOW IS THAT FEELING SERVING YOU? HOW MUCH OF YOUR DAY WAS SPENT THINKING ABOUT FOOD? WHAT IS AN EMOTION OR SITUATION CONNECTED WITH YOUR FOOD THAT YOU NEED TO LET GO OF TODAY?

DITCH THE DIET LIFE

_____ DAY OF _____, 20____

WORKOUT: MEDITATION TIME:

BREAKFAST:

LUNCH:

DINNER:

SNACKS:

ALCOHOL: YES OR NO. HOW MUCH

ON A SCALE OF 1-10, HOW WOULD YOUR RATE YOUR DAY?

DID YOU EXPERIENCE ANY PHYSICAL REACTIONS TO SOMETHING YOU ATE?

WHAT WAS THE BEST THING ABOUT YOUR DAY?
WHAT ARE YOU GRATEFUL FOR?

WATER CHECK: 1   2   3   4   5   6   7   8

Ditch the Diet Life ~ Brittnae Giesau

FREE WRITE

_____ DAY OF _____, 20___.

HERE ARE SOME QUESTIONS TO ASK YOURSELF:
DID YOU FEEL ANY GUILT AFTER EATING SOMETHING TODAY? HOW IS THAT FEELING SERVING YOU? HOW MUCH OF YOUR DAY WAS SPENT THINKING ABOUT FOOD? WHAT IS AN EMOTION OR SITUATION CONNECTED WITH YOUR FOOD THAT YOU NEED TO LET GO OF TODAY?

DITCH THE DIET LIFE

_____ DAY OF _____, 20____

WORKOUT: MEDITATION TIME:

BREAKFAST:

LUNCH:

DINNER:

SNACKS:

ALCOHOL: YES OR NO, HOW MUCH

ON A SCALE OF 1-10, HOW WOULD YOUR RATE YOUR DAY?

DID YOU EXPERIENCE ANY PHYSICAL REACTIONS TO SOMETHING YOU ATE?

WHAT WAS THE BEST THING ABOUT YOUR DAY?
WHAT ARE YOU GRATEFUL FOR?

WATER CHECK: 1   2   3   4   5   6   7   8

Ditch the Diet Life - Brittnae Giesau

FREE WRITE

_____ DAY OF _____, 20___.

HERE ARE SOME QUESTIONS TO ASK YOURSELF:
DID YOU FEEL ANY GUILT AFTER EATING SOMETHING TODAY? HOW IS THAT FEELING SERVING YOU? HOW MUCH OF YOUR DAY WAS SPENT THINKING ABOUT FOOD? WHAT IS AN EMOTION OR SITUATION CONNECTED WITH YOUR FOOD THAT YOU NEED TO LET GO OF TODAY?

Ditch the Diet Life ~ Brittnae Giesau

DITCH THE DIET LIFE

_____ DAY OF _____, 20____

WORKOUT: MEDITATION TIME:

BREAKFAST:

LUNCH:

DINNER:

SNACKS:

ALCOHOL: YES OR NO, HOW MUCH

ON A SCALE OF 1-10, HOW WOULD YOUR RATE YOUR DAY?

DID YOU EXPERIENCE ANY PHYSICAL REACTIONS TO SOMETHING YOU ATE?

WHAT WAS THE BEST THING ABOUT YOUR DAY? WHAT ARE YOU GRATEFUL FOR?

WATER CHECK: 1 2 3 4 5 6 7 8

Ditch the Diet Life ~ Brittnae Giesau

FREE WRITE

_____ DAY OF _____, 20___.

HERE ARE SOME QUESTIONS TO ASK YOURSELF:
DID YOU FEEL ANY GUILT AFTER EATING SOMETHING TODAY? HOW IS THAT FEELING SERVING YOU? HOW MUCH OF YOUR DAY WAS SPENT THINKING ABOUT FOOD? WHAT IS AN EMOTION OR SITUATION CONNECTED WITH YOUR FOOD THAT YOU NEED TO LET GO OF TODAY?

Ditch the Diet Life ~ Brittnae Giesau

DITCH THE DIET LIFE

_____ DAY OF _____, 20____

WORKOUT: MEDITATION TIME:

BREAKFAST:

LUNCH:

DINNER:

SNACKS:

ALCOHOL: YES OR NO, HOW MUCH

ON A SCALE OF 1-10, HOW WOULD YOUR RATE YOUR DAY?

DID YOU EXPERIENCE ANY PHYSICAL REACTIONS TO SOMETHING YOU ATE?

WHAT WAS THE BEST THING ABOUT YOUR DAY?
WHAT ARE YOU GRATEFUL FOR?

WATER CHECK: 1 2 3 4 5 6 7 8

Ditch the Diet Life ~ Brittnae Giesau

FREE WRITE

_____ DAY OF _____, 20___.

HERE ARE SOME QUESTIONS TO ASK YOURSELF:
DID YOU FEEL ANY GUILT AFTER EATING SOMETHING TODAY? HOW IS THAT FEELING SERVING YOU? HOW MUCH OF YOUR DAY WAS SPENT THINKING ABOUT FOOD? WHAT IS AN EMOTION OR SITUATION CONNECTED WITH YOUR FOOD THAT YOU NEED TO LET GO OF TODAY?

DITCH THE DIET LIFE

_____ DAY OF _____, 20____

WORKOUT: MEDITATION TIME:

BREAKFAST:

LUNCH:

DINNER:

SNACKS:

ALCOHOL: YES OR NO. HOW MUCH

ON A SCALE OF 1-10, HOW WOULD YOUR RATE YOUR DAY?

DID YOU EXPERIENCE ANY PHYSICAL REACTIONS TO SOMETHING YOU ATE?

WHAT WAS THE BEST THING ABOUT YOUR DAY?
WHAT ARE YOU GRATEFUL FOR?

WATER CHECK: 1 2 3 4 5 6 7 8

Ditch the Diet Life ~ Brittnae Giesau

FREE WRITE

_____ DAY OF _____, 20___.

HERE ARE SOME QUESTIONS TO ASK YOURSELF:
DID YOU FEEL ANY GUILT AFTER EATING SOMETHING TODAY? HOW IS THAT FEELING SERVING YOU? HOW MUCH OF YOUR DAY WAS SPENT THINKING ABOUT FOOD? WHAT IS AN EMOTION OR SITUATION CONNECTED WITH YOUR FOOD THAT YOU NEED TO LET GO OF TODAY?

Ditch the Diet Life ~ Brittnae Giesau

DITCH THE DIET LIFE

_____ DAY OF _____, 20____

WORKOUT: MEDITATION TIME:

BREAKFAST:

LUNCH:

DINNER:

SNACKS:

ALCOHOL: YES OR NO. HOW MUCH

ON A SCALE OF 1-10, HOW WOULD YOUR RATE YOUR DAY?

DID YOU EXPERIENCE ANY PHYSICAL REACTIONS TO SOMETHING YOU ATE?

WHAT WAS THE BEST THING ABOUT YOUR DAY? WHAT ARE YOU GRATEFUL FOR?

WATER CHECK: 1   2   3   4   5   6   7   8

Ditch the Diet Life ~ Brittnae Giesau

FREE WRITE

_____ DAY OF _____, 20___.

HERE ARE SOME QUESTIONS TO ASK YOURSELF:
DID YOU FEEL ANY GUILT AFTER EATING SOMETHING TODAY? HOW IS THAT FEELING SERVING YOU? HOW MUCH OF YOUR DAY WAS SPENT THINKING ABOUT FOOD? WHAT IS AN EMOTION OR SITUATION CONNECTED WITH YOUR FOOD THAT YOU NEED TO LET GO OF TODAY?

DITCH THE DIET LIFE

_____ DAY OF _____, 20____

WORKOUT: MEDITATION TIME:

BREAKFAST:

LUNCH:

DINNER:

SNACKS:

ALCOHOL: YES OR NO. HOW MUCH

ON A SCALE OF 1-10, HOW WOULD YOUR RATE YOUR DAY?

DID YOU EXPERIENCE ANY PHYSICAL REACTIONS TO SOMETHING YOU ATE?

WHAT WAS THE BEST THING ABOUT YOUR DAY?
WHAT ARE YOU GRATEFUL FOR?

WATER CHECK: 1   2   3   4   5   6   7   8

Ditch the Diet Life ~ Brittnae Giesau

FREE WRITE

_____ DAY OF _____, 20___.

HERE ARE SOME QUESTIONS TO ASK YOURSELF:
DID YOU FEEL ANY GUILT AFTER EATING SOMETHING TODAY? HOW IS THAT FEELING SERVING YOU? HOW MUCH OF YOUR DAY WAS SPENT THINKING ABOUT FOOD? WHAT IS AN EMOTION OR SITUATION CONNECTED WITH YOUR FOOD THAT YOU NEED TO LET GO OF TODAY?

DITCH THE DIET LIFE

_____ DAY OF _____, 20____

WORKOUT: MEDITATION TIME:

BREAKFAST:

LUNCH:

DINNER:

SNACKS:

ALCOHOL: YES OR NO. HOW MUCH

ON A SCALE OF 1-10, HOW WOULD YOUR RATE YOUR DAY?

DID YOU EXPERIENCE ANY PHYSICAL REACTIONS TO SOMETHING YOU ATE?

WHAT WAS THE BEST THING ABOUT YOUR DAY?
WHAT ARE YOU GRATEFUL FOR?

WATER CHECK: 1 2 3 4 5 6 7 8

Ditch the Diet Life ~ Brittnae Giesau

FREE WRITE

_____ DAY OF _____, 20___.

HERE ARE SOME QUESTIONS TO ASK YOURSELF:
DID YOU FEEL ANY GUILT AFTER EATING SOMETHING TODAY? HOW IS THAT FEELING SERVING YOU? HOW MUCH OF YOUR DAY WAS SPENT THINKING ABOUT FOOD? WHAT IS AN EMOTION OR SITUATION CONNECTED WITH YOUR FOOD THAT YOU NEED TO LET GO OF TODAY?

Ditch the Diet Life ~ Brittnae Giesau

To love oneself

is the beginning

of a lifelong

Romance.

DIGGING DEEPER

By now you should be learning a few things about yourself. For example: what foods you enjoy eating on a regular basis, how meditation might be helping you get more sleep at night, are you experiencing any patterns associated with eating in front of the television...

Remember, this is a process that takes time and one of the most important things that you can do is to give yourself grace. We tend to jump to judgment very quickly; Judgment of the foods that we eat, judgment of the feelings that we had before or after the food, or judgment of others because they're not on the same path as we are. Releasing your judgments, releases guilt & shame associated with food.

Light a candle, pour a glass of wine or sparkling water, grab your pen and take some time on the "making peace with food" & "writing deeper" sections on the next pages before moving on. These questions are not meant to scare you or for you to label food. Categorizing these foods allows you to be honest with how these foods may be triggering you.

Tomorrow you're going to see the same tracking sheet as you have had since you started, but your free write questions are going to change a bit. I would love to see you focus on the transition from trigger foods to safe foods through your free write each day, making peace with your food and taking a huge step towards ditching your diet life.

Don't forget to utilize the online support by joining our private Facebook community at facebook.com/groups/ditchdietlife.

MAKING PEACE WITH FOOD

"SAFE" FOODS: Any foods that you can enjoy free of emotional attachments or binge eating patterns.

"SCARY" FOODS: Any foods that you can eat with "safe boundaries" (i.e. not eating after a certain time, only having one)

"TRIGGER" FOODS: Any foods you tend to binge on or find yourself having negative emotions after eating so you try to abstain.

What are your "SAFE" foods?

What are your "SCARY" foods?

What are your "TRIGGER" foods?

*Remember there are no "scary" or "bad" foods. Words like safe, scary, bad, and trigger foods are only words that we attach our own emotions to the food. We are working to free you from these words.

WRITING DEEPER

HOW CAN YOU SET TEMPORARY BOUNDARIES
FOR YOUR TRIGGER FOODS TO MAKE THEM SCARY FOODS?

HOW CAN YOUR SCARY FOODS BECOME SAFE FOODS SO THAT ALL FOOD IS "SAFE"?

WHAT HAS BEEN THE BIGGEST OBSTACLE YOU HAVE
OVERCOME SINCE BEGINNING THIS PROCESS?

WRITE ABOUT ONE SITUATION IN THE LAST WEEK WHEN YOU USED YOUR
PRACTICES & FELT "FREE" FROM A DIET MENTALITY

DITCH THE DIET LIFE

_____ DAY OF _____, 20____

WORKOUT: MEDITATION TIME:

BREAKFAST:

LUNCH:

DINNER:

SNACKS:

ALCOHOL: YES OR NO. HOW MUCH

ON A SCALE OF 1-10, HOW WOULD YOUR RATE YOUR DAY?

DID YOU EXPERIENCE ANY PHYSICAL REACTIONS TO SOMETHING YOU ATE?

WHAT WAS THE BEST THING ABOUT YOUR DAY? WHAT ARE YOU GRATEFUL FOR?

WATER CHECK: 1 2 3 4 5 6 7 8

FREE WRITE

_____ DAY OF _____, 20___.

HERE ARE SOME QUESTIONS TO ASK YOURSELF:
DID YOU TEST YOURSELF WITH A TRIGGER OR SCARY FOOD TODAY? HOW DID THAT MAKE YOU FEEL? HOW CAN YOU TURN THOSE FEELINGS INTO POSITIVE TO TAKE A STEP TOWARDS THAT FOOD GOING ON THE SAFE FOOD CATEGORY? WHAT DID YOU FEEL OR SEE DURING MEDITATION TODAY?

Ditch the Diet Life ~ Brittnae Giesau

DITCH THE DIET LIFE

_____ DAY OF _____, 20___

WORKOUT: MEDITATION TIME:

BREAKFAST:

LUNCH:

DINNER:

SNACKS:

ALCOHOL: YES OR NO, HOW MUCH

ON A SCALE OF 1-10, HOW WOULD YOUR RATE YOUR DAY?

DID YOU EXPERIENCE ANY PHYSICAL REACTIONS TO SOMETHING YOU ATE?

WHAT WAS THE BEST THING ABOUT YOUR DAY?
WHAT ARE YOU GRATEFUL FOR?

WATER CHECK: 1 2 3 4 5 6 7 8

Ditch the Diet Life ~ Brittnae Giesau

FREE WRITE

_____ DAY OF _____, 20___.

HERE ARE SOME QUESTIONS TO ASK YOURSELF:
DID YOU TEST YOURSELF WITH A TRIGGER OR SCARY FOOD TODAY? HOW DID THAT MAKE YOU FEEL? HOW CAN YOU TURN THOSE FEELINGS INTO POSITIVE TO TAKE A STEP TOWARDS THAT FOOD GOING ON THE SAFE FOOD CATEGORY? WHAT DID YOU FEEL OR SEE DURING MEDITATION TODAY?

DITCH THE DIET LIFE

_____ DAY OF _____, 20____

WORKOUT: MEDITATION TIME:

BREAKFAST:

LUNCH:

DINNER:

SNACKS:

ALCOHOL: YES OR NO, HOW MUCH

ON A SCALE OF 1-10, HOW WOULD YOUR RATE YOUR DAY?

DID YOU EXPERIENCE ANY PHYSICAL REACTIONS TO SOMETHING YOU ATE?

WHAT WAS THE BEST THING ABOUT YOUR DAY?
WHAT ARE YOU GRATEFUL FOR?

WATER CHECK: 1 2 3 4 5 6 7 8

Ditch the Diet Life ~ Brittnae Giesau

FREE WRITE

_____ DAY OF _____, 20___.

HERE ARE SOME QUESTIONS TO ASK YOURSELF:
DID YOU TEST YOURSELF WITH A TRIGGER OR SCARY FOOD TODAY? HOW DID THAT MAKE YOU FEEL? HOW CAN YOU TURN THOSE FEELINGS INTO POSITIVE TO TAKE A STEP TOWARDS THAT FOOD GOING ON THE SAFE FOOD CATEGORY? WHAT DID YOU FEEL OR SEE DURING MEDITATION TODAY?

DITCH THE DIET LIFE

_____ DAY OF _____, 20___

WORKOUT: MEDITATION TIME:

BREAKFAST:

LUNCH:

DINNER:

SNACKS:

ALCOHOL: YES OR NO, HOW MUCH

ON A SCALE OF 1-10, HOW WOULD YOUR RATE YOUR DAY?

DID YOU EXPERIENCE ANY PHYSICAL REACTIONS TO SOMETHING YOU ATE?

WHAT WAS THE BEST THING ABOUT YOUR DAY?
WHAT ARE YOU GRATEFUL FOR?

WATER CHECK: 1 2 3 4 5 6 7 8

Ditch the Diet Life ~ Brittnae Giesau

FREE WRITE

_____ DAY OF _____, 20___.

HERE ARE SOME QUESTIONS TO ASK YOURSELF:
DID YOU TEST YOURSELF WITH A TRIGGER OR SCARY FOOD TODAY? HOW DID THAT MAKE YOU FEEL? HOW CAN YOU TURN THOSE FEELINGS INTO POSITIVE TO TAKE A STEP TOWARDS THAT FOOD GOING ON THE SAFE FOOD CATEGORY? WHAT DID YOU FEEL OR SEE DURING MEDITATION TODAY?

DITCH THE DIET LIFE

_____ DAY OF _____, 20___

WORKOUT: MEDITATION TIME:

BREAKFAST:

LUNCH:

DINNER:

SNACKS:

ALCOHOL: YES OR NO, HOW MUCH

ON A SCALE OF 1-10, HOW WOULD YOUR RATE YOUR DAY?

DID YOU EXPERIENCE ANY PHYSICAL REACTIONS TO SOMETHING YOU ATE?

WHAT WAS THE BEST THING ABOUT YOUR DAY?
WHAT ARE YOU GRATEFUL FOR?

WATER CHECK: 1 2 3 4 5 6 7 8

Ditch the Diet Life ~ Brittnae Giesau

FREE WRITE

_____ DAY OF _____, 20___.

HERE ARE SOME QUESTIONS TO ASK YOURSELF:
DID YOU TEST YOURSELF WITH A TRIGGER OR SCARY FOOD TODAY? HOW DID THAT MAKE YOU FEEL? HOW CAN YOU TURN THOSE FEELINGS INTO POSITIVE TO TAKE A STEP TOWARDS THAT FOOD GOING ON THE SAFE FOOD CATEGORY? WHAT DID YOU FEEL OR SEE DURING MEDITATION TODAY?

Ditch the Diet Life - Brittnae Giesau

DITCH THE DIET LIFE

_____ DAY OF _____, 20___

WORKOUT: MEDITATION TIME:

BREAKFAST:

LUNCH:

DINNER:

SNACKS:

ALCOHOL: YES OR NO, HOW MUCH

ON A SCALE OF 1-10, HOW WOULD YOUR RATE YOUR DAY?

DID YOU EXPERIENCE ANY PHYSICAL REACTIONS TO SOMETHING YOU ATE?

WHAT WAS THE BEST THING ABOUT YOUR DAY?
WHAT ARE YOU GRATEFUL FOR?

WATER CHECK: 1 2 3 4 5 6 7 8

Ditch the Diet Life ~ Brittnae Giesau

FREE WRITE

_____ DAY OF _____, 20___.

HERE ARE SOME QUESTIONS TO ASK YOURSELF:
DID YOU TEST YOURSELF WITH A TRIGGER OR SCARY FOOD TODAY? HOW DID THAT MAKE YOU FEEL? HOW CAN YOU TURN THOSE FEELINGS INTO POSITIVE TO TAKE A STEP TOWARDS THAT FOOD GOING ON THE SAFE FOOD CATEGORY? WHAT DID YOU FEEL OR SEE DURING MEDITATION TODAY?

DITCH THE DIET LIFE

_____ DAY OF _____, 20___

WORKOUT: MEDITATION TIME:

BREAKFAST:

LUNCH:

DINNER:

SNACKS:

ALCOHOL: YES OR NO, HOW MUCH

ON A SCALE OF 1-10, HOW WOULD YOUR RATE YOUR DAY?

DID YOU EXPERIENCE ANY PHYSICAL REACTIONS TO SOMETHING YOU ATE?

WHAT WAS THE BEST THING ABOUT YOUR DAY?
WHAT ARE YOU GRATEFUL FOR?

WATER CHECK: 1 2 3 4 5 6 7 8

Ditch the Diet Life ~ Brittnae Giesau

FREE WRITE

_____ DAY OF _____, 20___.

HERE ARE SOME QUESTIONS TO ASK YOURSELF:
DID YOU TEST YOURSELF WITH A TRIGGER OR SCARY FOOD TODAY? HOW DID THAT MAKE YOU FEEL? HOW CAN YOU TURN THOSE FEELINGS INTO POSITIVE TO TAKE A STEP TOWARDS THAT FOOD GOING ON THE SAFE FOOD CATEGORY? WHAT DID YOU FEEL OR SEE DURING MEDITATION TODAY?

DITCH THE DIET LIFE

_____ DAY OF _____, 20____

WORKOUT: MEDITATION TIME:

BREAKFAST:

LUNCH:

DINNER:

SNACKS:

ALCOHOL: YES OR NO, HOW MUCH

ON A SCALE OF 1-10, HOW WOULD YOUR RATE YOUR DAY?

DID YOU EXPERIENCE ANY PHYSICAL REACTIONS TO SOMETHING YOU ATE?

WHAT WAS THE BEST THING ABOUT YOUR DAY?
WHAT ARE YOU GRATEFUL FOR?

WATER CHECK: 1 2 3 4 5 6 7 8

FREE WRITE

_____ DAY OF _____, 20___.

HERE ARE SOME QUESTIONS TO ASK YOURSELF:
DID YOU TEST YOURSELF WITH A TRIGGER OR SCARY FOOD TODAY? HOW DID THAT MAKE YOU FEEL? HOW CAN YOU TURN THOSE FEELINGS INTO POSITIVE TO TAKE A STEP TOWARDS THAT FOOD GOING ON THE SAFE FOOD CATEGORY? WHAT DID YOU FEEL OR SEE DURING MEDITATION TODAY?

DITCH THE DIET LIFE

_____ DAY OF _____, 20____

WORKOUT: MEDITATION TIME:

BREAKFAST:

LUNCH:

DINNER:

SNACKS:

ALCOHOL: YES OR NO, HOW MUCH

ON A SCALE OF 1-10, HOW WOULD YOUR RATE YOUR DAY?

DID YOU EXPERIENCE ANY PHYSICAL REACTIONS TO SOMETHING YOU ATE?

WHAT WAS THE BEST THING ABOUT YOUR DAY?
WHAT ARE YOU GRATEFUL FOR?

WATER CHECK: 1 2 3 4 5 6 7 8

Ditch the Diet Life ~ Brittnae Giesau

FREE WRITE

_____ DAY OF _____, 20___.

HERE ARE SOME QUESTIONS TO ASK YOURSELF:
DID YOU TEST YOURSELF WITH A TRIGGER OR SCARY FOOD TODAY? HOW DID THAT MAKE YOU FEEL? HOW CAN YOU TURN THOSE FEELINGS INTO POSITIVE TO TAKE A STEP TOWARDS THAT FOOD GOING ON THE SAFE FOOD CATEGORY? WHAT DID YOU FEEL OR SEE DURING MEDITATION TODAY?

DITCH THE DIET LIFE

_____ DAY OF _____, 20____

WORKOUT: MEDITATION TIME:

BREAKFAST:

LUNCH:

DINNER:

SNACKS:

ALCOHOL: YES OR NO, HOW MUCH

ON A SCALE OF 1-10, HOW WOULD YOUR RATE YOUR DAY?

DID YOU EXPERIENCE ANY PHYSICAL REACTIONS TO SOMETHING YOU ATE?

WHAT WAS THE BEST THING ABOUT YOUR DAY?
WHAT ARE YOU GRATEFUL FOR?

WATER CHECK: 1   2   3   4   5   6   7   8

Ditch the Diet Life ~ Brittnae Giesau

FREE WRITE

_____ DAY OF _____, 20___.

HERE ARE SOME QUESTIONS TO ASK YOURSELF:
DID YOU TEST YOURSELF WITH A TRIGGER OR SCARY FOOD TODAY? HOW DID THAT MAKE YOU FEEL? HOW CAN YOU TURN THOSE FEELINGS INTO POSITIVE TO TAKE A STEP TOWARDS THAT FOOD GOING ON THE SAFE FOOD CATEGORY? WHAT DID YOU FEEL OR SEE DURING MEDITATION TODAY?

Self-Care isn't Selfish...

It's Necessary.

LOVE YOURSELF FIRST

Was that last section a little intense for you? It should have been. When we dig deeper into our mindset of how we truly feel about foods, we scare ourselves a little bit, but have a greater ability to create breakthroughs. It's time to lighten your load and work on taking care of and loving yourself.

Self-Care and Self-Love may seem to be overused on social media, but it's important to address. Women are nurturers by nature. We want to help everyone, fix everything, and take care of everyone else before ourselves. But when was the last time you said "no, I need to focus on me right now."

Self-Care is taking action and Self-Love is your emotion. The next section you will be focusing, not only on your diet mentality because we've done a lot of work on food mindset, but also taking time for yourself. This is an important step to wrap up your 30 days and I urge you not to skip through or brush it off.

Keep these exercises with you throughout the rest of the journal. The tracking sheets are the same as always, but again your free write will reflect this section. You have come so far already, and this is the fun part.

And because this is an incredibly important area for accountability, if you have not done so yet, please join our private community on Facebook at: facebook.com/groups/ditchdietlife.

SELF-CARE

Self-Care is the action of taking care of you. Practicing self-care is often looked upon as selfish or self-indulgent. Women are not wired to put themselves first. It's just not the nature of our gender. We want everyone to be happy and healthy and have everything they need, and if that comes at the expense of our own care, then so be it. But what would happen if for just one day (or 10 days as you're about to do) you focused on little things that would make you feel better? Chances are you will be happier, you will do your job better, your environment would be more peaceful, and you would be a better mom or wife. Self-Care isn't selfish, it's necessary.

Self-Care also means that sometimes you say no to things. You cannot be everything for everyone all the time. Saying no is scary because we worry how we are perceived or judged by others. But when we are practicing self-care, their opinions don't matter.

Self-Care doesn't need to be bubble baths and massages daily, or extravagant girls only vacations, or wearing pink fuzzy slippers sipping champagne in front of a roaring fire (though I'll take any of those any day!). Self-Care is sleeping in 5 or 10 minutes longer because you're comfy in your bed or cutting out a relationship with someone that isn't treating you the way you deserve or giving yourself grace when you've made a mistake instead of harboring guilt & resentment.

On the next page, I want you to think outside of your comfort zone. If there were no parameters, no meetings you have to attend at a certain time, no kids to run to a soccer practice, and the time was all yours, how would you take care of you?

PLANNING SELF-CARE

LIST 10 SELF-CARE ACTIVITIES THAT TAKE 10 MIN. OR LESS THAT YOU CAN BEGIN PRACTICING DAILY. (EX: 5 MIN. MORNING MEDITATION, COFFEE BEFORE ANYONE ELSE WAKES UP, MAKING YOUR BED, YOGA/STRETCHING, READ A CHAPTER OF A GOOD BOOK)

LIST 5 SELF-CARE ACTIVITIES THAT YOU LOVE TO DO, BUT DON'T MAKE TIME FOR, THAT YOU WILL SCHEDULE IN ONCE A WEEK. (EX: BUBBLE BATH, COFFEE DATE WITH A GIRLFRIEND, DATE NIGHT OUT WITH YOUR SPOUSE)

LIST 5 EMOTIONAL SELF-CARE SITUATIONS THAT YOU ARE STRUGGLING WITH AND COMMIT TO WORKING THROUGH. (EX: ROCKY FRIENDSHIPS, PROBLEMS AT WORK, FAMILY DISPUTES)

SELF-LOVE

Self-Love is the emotion that is built upon following your self-care actions. You cannot just make your bed, sip coffee quietly while reading a book and all of a sudden say "I love myself, my body is a temple". Self-Love takes emotional practice and is the underlying root of your diet mentality.

What kind of emotions do you attach to yourself when it comes to dieting? Do you have a positive or negative body image? Are you struggling to lose weight & grimace at the girl in the mirror every day? Or do you give yourself compliments or wear a sexy outfit to dinner or thank your body for being healthy & alive?

There's that time old lesson of "what you think, you are". It may seem silly, but it's the law of attraction. What you put out, you are going to receive. If you are staring in the mirror every single day picking apart each little dimple or roll or saggy spot, that's all you are ever going to see. If you stand in front of the mirror every day and find something new to love and be grateful for and remind that girl that she is beautiful, your body is going to be receptive.

On the next page you are going to write a letter to yourself. I encourage you to be more open and honest with yourself than ever before. Give gratitude for everything that your body has provided to you. Write, in detail, the most beautiful parts of your body. Tell her how you will love her and how you will honor her.

LETTER TO MYSELF

DITCH THE DIET LIFE

_____ DAY OF _____, 20____

WORKOUT: MEDITATION TIME:

BREAKFAST:

LUNCH:

DINNER:

SNACKS:

ALCOHOL: YES OR NO, HOW MUCH

ON A SCALE OF 1-10, HOW WOULD YOUR RATE YOUR DAY?

DID YOU EXPERIENCE ANY PHYSICAL REACTIONS TO SOMETHING YOU ATE?

WHAT WAS THE BEST THING ABOUT YOUR DAY?
WHAT ARE YOU GRATEFUL FOR?

WATER CHECK: 1 2 3 4 5 6 7 8

Ditch the Diet Life ~ Brittnae Giesau

FREE WRITE

_____ DAY OF _____, 20___.

HERE ARE SOME QUESTIONS TO ASK YOURSELF:
WHAT SELF-CARE ACTIVITIES DID YOU PRACTICE TODAY? WHAT ARE YOU LOVING ABOUT YOURSELF TODAY? DID ANY FOOD GUILT CREEP UP ON YOU? HOW IS THAT FEELING SERVING YOU? HOW CAN YOU RELEASE THAT FEELING?

Ditch the Diet Life ~ Brittnae Giesau

DITCH THE DIET LIFE

_____ DAY OF _____, 20____

WORKOUT: MEDITATION TIME:

BREAKFAST:

LUNCH:

DINNER:

SNACKS:

ALCOHOL: YES OR NO, HOW MUCH

ON A SCALE OF 1-10, HOW WOULD YOUR RATE YOUR DAY?

DID YOU EXPERIENCE ANY PHYSICAL REACTIONS TO SOMETHING YOU ATE?

WHAT WAS THE BEST THING ABOUT YOUR DAY?
WHAT ARE YOU GRATEFUL FOR?

WATER CHECK: 1 2 3 4 5 6 7 8

Ditch the Diet Life ~ Brittnae Giesau

FREE WRITE

_____ DAY OF _____, 20___.

HERE ARE SOME QUESTIONS TO ASK YOURSELF:
WHAT SELF-CARE ACTIVITIES DID YOU PRACTICE TODAY? WHAT ARE YOU LOVING ABOUT YOURSELF TODAY? DID ANY FOOD GUILT CREEP UP ON YOU? HOW IS THAT FEELING SERVING YOU? HOW CAN YOU RELEASE THAT FEELING?

DITCH THE DIET LIFE

_____ DAY OF _____, 20___

WORKOUT: MEDITATION TIME:

BREAKFAST:

LUNCH:

DINNER:

SNACKS:

ALCOHOL: YES OR NO, HOW MUCH

ON A SCALE OF 1-10, HOW WOULD YOUR RATE YOUR DAY?

DID YOU EXPERIENCE ANY PHYSICAL REACTIONS TO SOMETHING YOU ATE?

WHAT WAS THE BEST THING ABOUT YOUR DAY?
WHAT ARE YOU GRATEFUL FOR?

WATER CHECK: 1 2 3 4 5 6 7 8

Ditch the Diet Life ~ Brittnae Giesau

FREE WRITE

_____ DAY OF _____, 20___.

HERE ARE SOME QUESTIONS TO ASK YOURSELF:
WHAT SELF-CARE ACTIVITIES DID YOU PRACTICE TODAY? WHAT ARE YOU LOVING ABOUT YOURSELF TODAY? DID ANY FOOD GUILT CREEP UP ON YOU? HOW IS THAT FEELING SERVING YOU? HOW CAN YOU RELEASE THAT FEELING?

Ditch the Diet Life ~ Brittnae Giesau

DITCH THE DIET LIFE

_____ DAY OF _____, 20____

WORKOUT:

MEDITATION TIME:

BREAKFAST:

LUNCH:

DINNER:

SNACKS:

ALCOHOL: YES OR NO, HOW MUCH

ON A SCALE OF 1-10, HOW WOULD YOUR RATE YOUR DAY?

DID YOU EXPERIENCE ANY PHYSICAL REACTIONS TO SOMETHING YOU ATE?

WHAT WAS THE BEST THING ABOUT YOUR DAY?
WHAT ARE YOU GRATEFUL FOR?

WATER CHECK: 1 2 3 4 5 6 7 8

Ditch the Diet Life - Brittnae Giesau

FREE WRITE

_____ DAY OF _____, 20___.

HERE ARE SOME QUESTIONS TO ASK YOURSELF:
WHAT SELF-CARE ACTIVITIES DID YOU PRACTICE TODAY? WHAT ARE YOU LOVING ABOUT YOURSELF TODAY? DID ANY FOOD GUILT CREEP UP ON YOU? HOW IS THAT FEELING SERVING YOU? HOW CAN YOU RELEASE THAT FEELING?

DITCH THE DIET LIFE

_____ DAY OF _____, 20____

WORKOUT:

MEDITATION TIME:

BREAKFAST:

LUNCH:

DINNER:

SNACKS:

ALCOHOL: YES OR NO, HOW MUCH

ON A SCALE OF 1-10, HOW WOULD YOUR RATE YOUR DAY?

DID YOU EXPERIENCE ANY PHYSICAL REACTIONS TO SOMETHING YOU ATE?

WHAT WAS THE BEST THING ABOUT YOUR DAY?
WHAT ARE YOU GRATEFUL FOR?

WATER CHECK: 1 2 3 4 5 6 7 8

Ditch the Diet Life ~ Brittnae Giesau

FREE WRITE

_____ DAY OF _____, 20___.

HERE ARE SOME QUESTIONS TO ASK YOURSELF:
WHAT SELF-CARE ACTIVITIES DID YOU PRACTICE TODAY? WHAT ARE YOU LOVING ABOUT YOURSELF TODAY? DID ANY FOOD GUILT CREEP UP ON YOU? HOW IS THAT FEELING SERVING YOU? HOW CAN YOU RELEASE THAT FEELING?

DITCH THE DIET LIFE

_____ DAY OF _____, 20____

WORKOUT: MEDITATION TIME:

BREAKFAST:

LUNCH:

DINNER:

SNACKS:

ALCOHOL: YES OR NO, HOW MUCH

ON A SCALE OF 1-10, HOW WOULD YOUR RATE YOUR DAY?

DID YOU EXPERIENCE ANY PHYSICAL REACTIONS TO SOMETHING YOU ATE?

WHAT WAS THE BEST THING ABOUT YOUR DAY?
WHAT ARE YOU GRATEFUL FOR?

WATER CHECK: 1 2 3 4 5 6 7 8

Ditch the Diet Life ~ Brittnae Giesau

FREE WRITE

_____ DAY OF _____, 20___.

HERE ARE SOME QUESTIONS TO ASK YOURSELF:
WHAT SELF-CARE ACTIVITIES DID YOU PRACTICE TODAY? WHAT ARE YOU LOVING ABOUT YOURSELF TODAY? DID ANY FOOD GUILT CREEP UP ON YOU? HOW IS THAT FEELING SERVING YOU? HOW CAN YOU RELEASE THAT FEELING?

Ditch the Diet Life ~ Brittnae Giesau

DITCH THE DIET LIFE

_____ DAY OF _____, 20____

WORKOUT: MEDITATION TIME:

BREAKFAST:

LUNCH:

DINNER:

SNACKS:

ALCOHOL: YES OR NO, HOW MUCH

ON A SCALE OF 1-10, HOW WOULD YOUR RATE YOUR DAY?

DID YOU EXPERIENCE ANY PHYSICAL REACTIONS TO SOMETHING YOU ATE?

WHAT WAS THE BEST THING ABOUT YOUR DAY?
WHAT ARE YOU GRATEFUL FOR?

WATER CHECK: 1 2 3 4 5 6 7 8

Ditch the Diet Life ~ Brittnae Giesau

FREE WRITE

_____ DAY OF _____, 20___.

HERE ARE SOME QUESTIONS TO ASK YOURSELF:
WHAT SELF-CARE ACTIVITIES DID YOU PRACTICE TODAY? WHAT ARE YOU LOVING ABOUT YOURSELF TODAY? DID ANY FOOD GUILT CREEP UP ON YOU? HOW IS THAT FEELING SERVING YOU? HOW CAN YOU RELEASE THAT FEELING?

DITCH THE DIET LIFE

_____ DAY OF _____, 20____

WORKOUT: MEDITATION TIME:

BREAKFAST:

LUNCH:

DINNER:

SNACKS:

ALCOHOL: YES OR NO, HOW MUCH

ON A SCALE OF 1-10, HOW WOULD YOUR RATE YOUR DAY?

DID YOU EXPERIENCE ANY PHYSICAL REACTIONS TO SOMETHING YOU ATE?

WHAT WAS THE BEST THING ABOUT YOUR DAY?
WHAT ARE YOU GRATEFUL FOR?

WATER CHECK: 1 2 3 4 5 6 7 8

Ditch the Diet Life ~ Brittnae Giesau

FREE WRITE

_____ DAY OF _____, 20___.

HERE ARE SOME QUESTIONS TO ASK YOURSELF:
WHAT SELF-CARE ACTIVITIES DID YOU PRACTICE TODAY? WHAT ARE YOU LOVING ABOUT YOURSELF TODAY? DID ANY FOOD GUILT CREEP UP ON YOU? HOW IS THAT FEELING SERVING YOU? HOW CAN YOU RELEASE THAT FEELING?

DITCH THE DIET LIFE

_____ DAY OF _____, 20___

WORKOUT:

MEDITATION TIME:

BREAKFAST:

LUNCH:

DINNER:

SNACKS:

ALCOHOL: YES OR NO, HOW MUCH

ON A SCALE OF 1-10, HOW WOULD YOUR RATE YOUR DAY?

DID YOU EXPERIENCE ANY PHYSICAL REACTIONS TO SOMETHING YOU ATE?

WHAT WAS THE BEST THING ABOUT YOUR DAY?
WHAT ARE YOU GRATEFUL FOR?

WATER CHECK: 1 2 3 4 5 6 7 8

Ditch the Diet Life ~ Brittnae Giesau

FREE WRITE

_____ DAY OF _____, 20___.

HERE ARE SOME QUESTIONS TO ASK YOURSELF:
WHAT SELF-CARE ACTIVITIES DID YOU PRACTICE TODAY? WHAT ARE YOU LOVING ABOUT YOURSELF TODAY? DID ANY FOOD GUILT CREEP UP ON YOU? HOW IS THAT FEELING SERVING YOU? HOW CAN YOU RELEASE THAT FEELING?

Ditch the Diet Life ~ Brittnae Giesau

DITCH THE DIET LIFE

_____ DAY OF _____, 20____

WORKOUT: MEDITATION TIME:

BREAKFAST:

LUNCH:

DINNER:

SNACKS:

ALCOHOL: YES OR NO, HOW MUCH

ON A SCALE OF 1-10, HOW WOULD YOUR RATE YOUR DAY?

DID YOU EXPERIENCE ANY PHYSICAL REACTIONS TO SOMETHING YOU ATE?

WHAT WAS THE BEST THING ABOUT YOUR DAY?
WHAT ARE YOU GRATEFUL FOR?

WATER CHECK: 1 2 3 4 5 6 7 8

Ditch the Diet Life ~ Brittnae Giesau

FREE WRITE

_____ DAY OF _____, 20___.

HERE ARE SOME QUESTIONS TO ASK YOURSELF:
WHAT SELF-CARE ACTIVITIES DID YOU PRACTICE TODAY? WHAT ARE YOU LOVING ABOUT YOURSELF TODAY? DID ANY FOOD GUILT CREEP UP ON YOU? HOW IS THAT FEELING SERVING YOU? HOW CAN YOU RELEASE THAT FEELING?

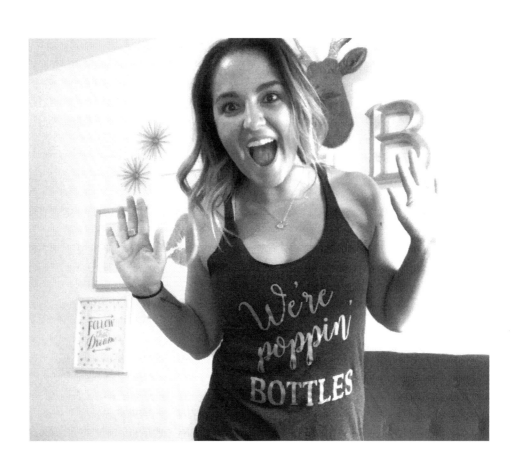

CONGRATULATIONS

You did it. You have completed 30 days of this journey. I am not going to tell you congratulations for ditching your diet life, because this is not the end. As I told you in the beginning of this workbook, this is a process. You may have had years of roller coaster diet struggles and emotional attachments with food and body image; it doesn't miraculously disappear in 30 days.

What you have done is built a foundation. You gave yourself this gift of taking your first steps, honoring yourself, and teaching your brain new habits and thoughts. Now it is time for you to take the next steps and be accountable to following the path to Ditch Your Diet Life. Diet mindsets are going to creep back all the time, it happens for me too. The difference is that you now have trained yourself to be aware of those thoughts and feelings and address them as they come to you. You can take these steps that we worked through in this journal into your day-to-day life and I hope that you do. If at any time you feel that you need a refresher, grab a clean workbook and join me again on this journey.

Thank you for letting me be a part of your journey and trusting me to guide you through these first steps. This is not the end for you, this is only the beginning. I wish you all of the love and support that I can give you to end your dieting mentality for good.

You are worth it. You deserve it. You will ditch it.

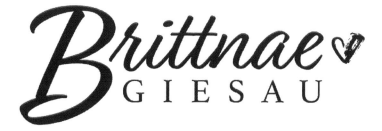

Made in the USA
Monee, IL
25 February 2020